The IDEAL You

5 SECRETS TO ACHIEVING YOUR GOAL WEIGHT

By Dr. Henry Wong, DC

TABLE OF CONTENTS

CHAPTER ONE

WHY WEIGHT LOSS?

The topic of weight loss seems to be everywhere you turn. It feels like you can't even turn on the television anymore without seeing someone talking about ways you can lose weight. Why is this such a prominent topic in the 21st century? There is one simple reason for all the fuss surrounding the topic of weight loss –

America is fat.

Harsh, but true. The stats don't lie, and they are staggering. According to research performed by the U.S. Department of Health in 2017, nearly 40% of American adults are considered obese. By any measure, that is an epidemic, and it keeps getting worse. Perhaps even more troubling is the fact that almost 20% of adolescents are considered obese, which is the worst number in recorded history. Not only are the current numbers incredibly disturbing, the trend of weight gain over time indicates that this problem is going to get worse before it gets better. Unless radical changes are made, Americans are going to keep getting bigger and bigger, and sicker and sicker.

So, what is the problem? As is usually the case with a problem this large, there is more than one underlying cause at the heart of this issue.

Whenever the topic of obesity and weight loss is on the table, there are generally two main factors which need to be addressed.

- Diet. Of course, this is where it all starts. When people eat too much – and eat too much of the wrong kinds of foods – they gain weight. You don't need to be a dietician to understand the link between what goes into your mouth and what happens on the scale. If you eat a bad diet, you are almost certainly going to gain weight over time. On the other hand, you will have an excellent chance to maintain a healthy weight if you eat a balanced diet composed mostly of fruits and vegetables. The food you provide your body is the fuel that your body uses to operate each day. Give yourself quality fuel, and your body will work as it is intended to work.

Provide poor fuel, however, and all bets are off.

- Exercise. While diet is certainly the main culprit with regard to the obesity epidemic, exercise has a role to play as well. With the rise of modern technology, Americans – and many others around the world – are living an increasingly sedentary lifestyle. Jobs that used to require manual labor are now performed at desks in many cases, taking built-in exercise away from the employee. Unless you happen to have one of the remaining manual labor jobs in the modern workforce, you will need to get your exercise elsewhere. And, sadly, for most people, that simply doesn't happen. Millions of people go throughout their day simply moving from one sitting position to the next. If you think about your average day, there is a good chance that the vast majority of it is spent sitting or lying down. You wake up in the morning after sleeping all night, quickly get ready for your day, and then sit back down in your car. After commuting to work in your car, you walk into the office and sit down again. You sit for the majority of the next eight hours, before sitting back down in your car for the drive home. After sitting down for dinner, you settle into the couch for a few TV shows before bed. If this routine sounds anything like your own, you are spending very little time during the average day getting any form of physical exercise. When this stationary lifestyle is combined with a poor diet, the results are all too predictable.

This two-headed monster has led to the record obesity rates that we discussed earlier. Without intervention on both of these fronts, the problem is just going to get worse. In this book, we hope to shed some light on how individuals can turn their weight problem around by taking action. It is easy to get swept along with everyone else in the trend of eating more and moving less – but you do have a choice in the matter. If you decide to make a change, it just may be the best change you've ever made.

The bulk of this book is going to be dedicated to helping you get back on track. However, before we get into that discussion, we first need to take an even closer look at how we wound up here in the first place.

The SAD Diet

In this case, SAD stands for 'Standard American Diet', and it certainly is a sad story. The average American has gotten so far away from the basics of good nutrition that they can't even imagine finding their way back. Most people today get by on a combination of fast food, prepackaged food from the grocery store, and sugary snacks. The ability to prepare a healthy meal at home is something that simply isn't possessed by a large percentage of the population.

You can probably take an honest look at your own diet and see many of the negative trends that are common across the country. Do you eat fresh fruits and vegetables on a regular basis? How many whole grains do you consume each day? Most likely, you are coming up short in these categories. It is actually quite rare for an American today to consume the appropriate amount of fruits, vegetables, and grains.

On the other hand, there are some categories where your consumption is likely off the charts. We can start with meat. It is estimated that more than 30% of American calories are consumed in the form of animal protein, which is almost certainly a number that should be much, much lower. On the other hand, barely more than 10% of calories are coming from whole grains, fruits, vegetables, and nuts. This is where most of your calories should be coming from, but that simply is not the case for most people.

A Problem for the Future

The present-day obesity problem is a substantial one, to say the least. More concerning, however, is what it means for the future. With more kids falling into the obese category than ever before, and the trend continuing to move in the wrong direction, what will the future look like for this generation? In addition to a bad diet, many of these kids are being brought up on video games and internet videos – not exactly a recipe for an active, healthy lifestyle.

Of course, a major issue with regard to obesity in children is the fact that they are simply following the lead set for them by their parents. If the parents eat an unhealthy diet, the kids are likely to do the same. If the parents lead a stationary lifestyle, the kids will be prone to sit around all day as well. Without a doubt, the transformation that needs to take place with children's health is going to have to start at the top. When parents begin to lead a healthy lifestyle, their kids are going to be very likely to follow along.

The Connection Between Weight Gain and Health Problems

One of the common misconceptions in the world of weight loss is that losing weight is all about looking good. Some people make the mistake of thinking that if they aren't concerned about their appearance, they shouldn't be too worried about their weight, either. Nothing could be further from the truth. While some people might stay in shape for vanity purposes, maintaining a healthy weight is more about your overall health than anything else.

So, what kind of health conditions can come about as a result of being overweight or obese? Let's look at a partial list:

- High blood pressure
- Diabetes
- Heart disease
- Stroke

- Some forms of cancer
- And on and on

If you can think of a serious disease, there is a good chance that your risk of obtaining that disease will be increased when you carry too much weight. There are other factors at play with many of these diseases, of course, but being obese is only going to turn the odds against you moving forward. Those who are able to maintain a healthy weight, or lose enough weight to fall into a healthy range, will stand a far better chance at remaining healthy for years to come.

The job of caring for your health starts at home. Sure, it is a good idea to turn to a medical professional when you have a condition that needs to be addressed, but your care should start with you managing a balanced diet and plenty of exercise. If you can hit on those two points on your own, it is going to be much easier for your doctor to do his or her job in terms of offering treatment.

Current 'Solutions' Are Not Working

As you know, there are plenty of solutions out there on the market today for you to consider. If you have a weight problem, you have already noticed the advertisements that come at you from every angle – on TV, on the radio, on the web, and beyond. America is a capitalist marketplace, and there is no shortage of products and services hoping to cash in on the obesity epidemic.

Should you turn to one of these solutions for help? Probably not. After all, if these options work, why do we still have such a problem with obesity in this country? While some of the options on the market might work for a percentage of the population, you aren't likely to have great results when chasing one magic solution after the next.

Diet plans and diet pills are two of the biggest potential solutions that people turn to for help. Unfortunately, neither of these are likely to hold up over the long run. For one thing, diet pills can be dangerous, and there is very little evidence to prove their effectiveness. At best, you are probably wasting money when you purchase diet pills, and at worst you may even be harming your health.

When it comes to diet plans, the company selling the plan usually has something else to sell you – a diet food of some kind. Those foods, while low in calories, also tend to be devoid of any real nutritional value. They might taste okay in some cases, but that is usually because they are loaded with salt and preservatives. Far from healthy, they just attempt to momentarily fill you up with fake food. If you have the willpower, you might be able to lose a few pounds while basically starving yourself of the nutrition that your body desires. Over the long run, however, this method is almost certain to fall short. You'll return to the foods you used to eat, and your weight will return, as well.

Looking Forward

So, is all hope lost with regard to finding a healthy weight in your future? Absolutely not. The key here is to ignore all of the marketing fluff and just listen to what your body needs. The body is designed to function in a specific way, and if you can supply your body with what it is looking for, you should be able to settle on a weight that is appropriate for your body type. Sure, there might be some hard work required at first to make the necessary changes, but you will be glad you put in the work when you see the progress you have made weeks and months down the line.

The title I.D.E.A.L represents five keys that we want to highlight in this book. Those five points are as follows –

- Inflammation and Iodine
- Detoxification
- Essential Vitamins & Minerals
- Acidity/Alkalization
- Low (or imbalanced) Hormones

As you will see in the content to follow, each of these points plays an important role in your overall health. As important as it is, remember, this is not just about finding a healthy weight. You also want to find an overall level of fitness that allows you to lead the lifestyle you would like to enjoy.

Up until this point, we have been looking at a lot of negative points. The obesity problem in America, the Standard American Diet (SAD) etc. From this point forward, however, we are going to turn in a positive direction. Rather than dwelling on what is wrong, we are going to get down to work on finding a way to fix the issues.

Let's get started!

INFLAMMATION AND IODINE

At first, it might seem a bit strange to start off a book about weight loss with inflammation and iodine but these are the 2 most commonly overlooked areas when it comes to identifying the causes of weight gain. After all, you've probably only heard of inflammation when you get hurt and when the body is healing but no one seems to relate to it when it comes to losing weight. The same is true for iodine. Most people never think about their iodine levels in any capacity, let alone in regard to their weight. This is why we would like to introduce you to the importance of these 2 elements, and explain why they need to be addressed in order for you to lose weight.

Let's talk about Inflammation first.

As mentioned earlier, we are familiar with inflammation when we're hurt. This is called "acute inflammation" where if you stub your toe or you get a cut or a burn, or maybe a black eye, your body's natural inflammatory response is redness, warmth, swelling and even loss of function. This acute inflammation is necessary and is your body's mechanism to help protect and heal itself – This is a good thing.

The second type, chronic inflammation, is different, scary and not a good thing. Especially because the symptoms aren't obvious like they are with acute inflammation. Chronic inflammation manifests itself in many ways from one person to another but it is the root cause of almost all weight gain and chronic disease and most all of us have it to some degree. In one person, inflammation may show up as heart disease, in another person as acne and in another as obesity. Chronic inflammation can contribute to a multitude of symptoms in the body such as achy joints, asthma, irritable bowel disease, diabetes, cancer, heart disease, migraines, skin rashes and the list goes on. Chronic inflammation is low grade and systemic, constantly engaged and silently damaging tissues and blocking you from reaching various health goals and increasing your risk of disease. You may not feel inflammation accumulating in your arteries but that doesn't mean you won't eventually suffer a heart attack.

Chronic inflammation is the kind that festers deep inside your tissues. Your body sees it as a fire and is always going to prioritize taking care of the inflammation before anything else. This means that if you're struggling with lack of energy, difficulty losing weight, or even digestive issues, it's going to be nearly impossible for your body to fix these issues without reducing inflammation first. Whether you want to lose weight or simply be healthier and at a lower risk for disease, we need to take care of this debilitating chronic inflammation.

In order to understand how to heal chronic inflammation, it's important to get to the root cause and understand how this problem developed in the first place. Chronic inflammation can be caused by things such as:

- Stress
- Smoking
- Overeating

- Poorly controlled diabetes
- Sugar
- Trans fats (anything fried or battered, pie crust, margarine, shortening, cake mix and frostings, pancakes, ice cream, non-dairy creamers, microwave popcorn, etc.)
- Processed Vegetable Oils (canola, soybean, corn, safflower, sunflower, palm etc.)
- Artificial Sweeteners
- Refined Carbohydrates (bread, pasta, cereal, crackers, and of course cookies, muffins and bagels)
- Excessive alcohol consumption
- Food Sensitivities
- Antibiotics in conventionally raised meat
- Lack of sleep

As you can see, most of these are lifestyle habits that YOU can personally manage. Who would have thought that sandwiches on whole grain bread could cause inflammation? Weren't we told that vegetable oils were healthy for our heart? And aren't artificial sweeteners supposed to be a better alternative to sugar? Let me explain: Eating foods that our body cannot process and embracing bad habits (like smoking, consuming excessive alcohol, not getting enough sleep, etc.) put a lot of stress on our body over time. Think of it as putting out little fires, except there is likely a fire going on all day every day if you are affected by any of the causes in the list above. In essence, your body is in a state of emergency all the time without you knowing or feeling it.

Food sensitivities, which are different for every person, also add to inflammation. If you are eating foods you have a sensitivity to, an inflammatory reaction takes place in your body and you are NOT going to lose weight. Your body is going to focus on healing areas that are affected (damaged and inflamed) by the food you are eating. This is why it is important to figure out what foods you may be more sensitive to. How much is too much? It's different for everyone, but you can bet that if you're doing too much of it and not giving your body a chance to rest, the physical stress you're putting on yourself won't be doing you any favors.

How can inflammation halt weight loss?

As we covered, inflammation sets the stage for a host of issues that affect your weight. If you have any inflammation going on in your body, the last thing your body will focus on is weight loss. Your body is designed to SURVIVE so it will want to take care of putting out all of the little fires your body is exposed to daily rather than shedding those pounds. Your body has its own list of priorities, and they may not be the same as yours. If you have lots of inflammation, trouble sleeping, have a hormone problem, or are too stressed out, your body is more interested in healing those issues than burning stored fat. If you learn to listen to your body, give it time, and nourish it with good, healing nutrition, it will thank you by shedding a few pounds once it is ready. The first step is healing the damage with real food and natural supplementation to get our bodies on the right track for weight loss.

Let's move onto Iodine.

The biggest job of iodine once it enters your body is to control the function of your thyroid gland. As you may know, the thyroid gland sits wrapped around the windpipe behind and below the Adam's Apple area and is largely responsible for the functioning of your hormone production and your metabolism.

This small bowtie-shaped gland produces several hormones in both men and women, the two most important being triiodothyronine (T3) and thyroxine (T4). These hormones help convert oxygen and calories into energy, making the thyroid the master gland of metabolism. These hormones are also essential for the proper functioning of all our organs, including our heart, musculoskeletal system and brain. Therefore, if your thyroid is not working up to capacity, it can cause your metabolism to slow and cause you to carry extra weight. It is safe to say that individuals who are deficient in iodine may run into problems with a sluggish thyroid gland which can then lead to weight gain as well as other problems like depression, fatigue, and more. Obviously, these symptoms will vary from person to person, but the research shows that the thyroid has a significant impact on your overall health.

According to the American Thyroid Association, there are an estimated 20 million Americans who have a thyroid disease and more than half are undiagnosed or even misdiagnosed, which is alarming. Why is this? One problem is that because symptoms of a sluggish thyroid (hypothyroidism) often vary from person to person and are non-specific, the correct diagnosis can easily be missed. Many cases remain undiagnosed because some practitioners and the patients themselves mistake the symptoms of hypothyroidism for depression, obesity or menopause.

Fortunately, it is not particularly difficult to find enough iodine in a healthy diet to improve the function of your thyroid gland. This mineral can be obtained in a variety of different healthy foods, meaning you will have plenty of choices when trying to add to your iodine intake. Some of the common ways to add iodine to your diet are listed below –

- Products of the sea, such as fish, seaweed, shrimp, etc.
- Iodized salt. It is easy to purchase iodized salt in the U.S., however the salt which is added to processed foods usually does not contain iodine.
- Dairy products and whole grain foods
- Fruits and vegetables, depending on the amount of iodine present in the soil where the plants grew before harvest

As you can see, the choices for adding iodine to your diet tend to be relatively healthy foods. While you don't want to overload your diet with salt – as it can have its own negative effects – using a little bit of iodized salt may be an effective way to add this valuable mineral to your meals. Of course, eating fruits and vegetables is always a good choice, and some fish are quite healthy for you, as well.

There are many potential health benefits which come along with iodine, including the following:

- Removal of toxins from the body
- Optimal utilization of calories
- Functioning of the thyroid (as mentioned above)
- Proper hormone production
- Proper metabolic function

Lacking iodine could cause your thyroid to underperform and can cause many symptoms including:

- Fatigue
- Difficulty losing weight
- A puffy face
- Trouble tolerating cold
- Joint and muscle pain
- Constipation

- Dry skin
- Dry, thinning hair
- Decreased sweating
- Heavy or irregular menstrual periods
- Fertility problems
- Depression
- Slowed heart rate
- Goiter

If you have one or more of these symptoms, it would be beneficial to monitor your overall diet and keep track of how many foods you consume which contain iodine. By doing this, you can be sure to avoid these potential health problems.

Supplementing your diet with an iodine rich supplement can also help tremendously. You will be doing yourself a favor in terms of maintaining a healthy weight by keeping your thyroid working at full capacity.

As with many of today's illnesses, the increased incidence of thyroid disease can be linked to an over-burden of toxins caused by pollution through air, water and food. If you have a concern about your thyroid, you may want to note that it may be due to being too toxic, which leads us to the next chapter – Detoxification.

CHAPTER THREE

DETOXIFICATION

There are a multitude of toxins that our bodies are exposed to everyday and being too toxic causes our bodies to become bogged down and not to be able to function at 100% capacity. Here is a list of the most common toxins that we expose our bodies to on a daily basis which can affect our thyroid gland and slow our metabolism –

- **Soy** - high soy consumers and users of isoflavone supplements can be at risk of thyroid disorders since soy isoflavones can damage thyroid function.

- **Smoking** – has a negative impact on thyroid function and can cause a 3 to 5 fold increase in the risk of all types of thyroid disease.
- **Tap water** - Standard water-treatment plants cannot remove the chemical perchlorate from the water supply. According to one researcher, "There is a statistical association between low-level contamination with ammonium perchlorate and elevated or abnormal thyroid function." Also, chlorine content in the water can displace the much-needed iodine.
- **Fluoride** – is an enzyme poison which accumulates in the body. Since the body can only eliminate 50% of its total fluoride intake, this build-up can cause harm to the thyroid by blocking the use of iodine.

- **Heavy metal** poisoning (as with mercury, lead, arsenic, and cadmium) of the thyroid can also lead to hypothyroidism; chemicals and pesticides can also be a factor.
- **Root canal teeth** can leak toxins into the body and enter the thyroid gland, producing malfunction.
- **Pesticides** - such as sumithrin (Anvil) and resmethrin (Scourge), are coming under considerable criticism for their adverse chronic effects on the thyroid.
- **Radiation and X-Rays** – are known to cause damage to the thyroid and other body parts.
- **Stress** – is a factor in almost every kind of disease and can affect the thyroid.
- **Toxic and Genetically Modified Foods (GMOs)**–Gluten allergies in particular cause disruptions to your thyroid function. GMOs cause many

health issues because the body doesn't process these genetically modified foods the same way as non-GMO foods. When corn, soy, or other foods are genetically modified, this will change the DNA, and the immune system sees the proteins in these foods as foreign. This triggers an immune system response, resulting in inflammation and erosion of the gut lining, which can lead to many different health issues including thyroid disease.

Each and every case is different though - some people find when they eliminate a certain food from their diet, their thyroid function stabilizes and their metabolism improves. The task is to identify which food groups are specifically toxic to your body. Speaking about food groups, let's spend some time and talk about real food.

How much real food do you eat? Stop and think about this question for a second. When you prepare your meals for the day, or you purchase meals from restaurants, how much of what you are putting into your body is real food? If you are anything like the average American, there is a good chance that you eat very little in the way of real food on a day to day basis.

We need to stop for a moment and explain what we mean by 'real' food. In this context, we consider real food to be something that has not been altered from its original state by chemicals, preservatives, additives, etc. For example, an apple that you simply purchase from the store and consume is a real food. On the other hand, a prepackage applesauce which has been filled up with sugar and preservatives would not be considered a real food (note: not all apple sauces are bad, but many of those found in the grocery store are unhealthy).

You can apply this line of thinking to just about everything you eat. As a basic rule of thumb, you want to eat the foods that have been altered the least by the time they land on your plate. In this way, you can work to detoxify your diet by taking out the things that nature probably never intended for you to consume. By eating more real food, and less and less of the fake stuff that fills the grocery store shelves, you will have a great opportunity to regain control of both your weight and your health.

To put the concept of detoxifying your diet into more practical terms, let's take a look at a few simple ideas that you can put into action.

- Start with snacks. Making changes in your snack foods is a great way to send your diet in a healthier direction. Often, snack foods are some of the biggest culprits in a poor diet, as they tend to be high in calories, low in nutrition, and filled with all sorts of chemicals and preservatives that you shouldn't be consuming. For example, let's say that you normally head to the vending machine at work for a late-afternoon snack. In most vending machines, you will find nothing but junk – thinks like chips, candy bars, etc. Most of the 'food' in a vending machine is either fried and salty, or all sugar. As a better option, think about taking a piece of fruit for your afternoon snack. By eating something like a banana, you will get some natural sugar, and you'll also get plenty of nutrients (and few calories). Even making this kind of simple switch can really help you take your diet in the right direction – and you can begin the process of removing toxins from your body.

- One scratch meal a week. If you are currently used to consuming mostly food that other people have prepared, it is going to be difficult to immediately switch to making all of your own food. With that said, you should work toward that goal by taking baby steps. For starters, try having one dinner per week that you make completely from scratch. That means no pre-made foods going into the meal, but starting from just plain ingredients like fruits, vegetables, lean proteins, spices, etc. You can use the internet as a powerful resource when learning how to cook meals from scratch, and you will find that these foods are deeply satisfying once you get the hang of it. Pretty soon, you'll become addicted to the feeling of creating your own meals and knowing exactly what is going into your body.

- Pay attention to color. One of the easiest ways to decide whether or not you are eating a healthy food is by looking at the color of that food. Is the food a natural shade, or does it look like it was developed in a lab? You don't need to have any kind of nutritional expertise to apply this eye test to the foods you pick out in the grocery store. A great example of this concept is the sugary cereals that so many people feed themselves – and their kids – every morning. These cereals are not only packed with sugar, but they are also full of artificial coloring. Those artificial colors have been linked to a long list of nasty diseases, including some cancers. You will be doing yourself a big favor if you can stay far away from foods which have had their colors modified artificially.

- Detoxing from excess sugar. Excessive sugar consumption is one of the biggest dietary problems in America today. And here's the thing – many people don't even know they are consuming nearly as much sugar as they are on a day to day basis.

- The problem is that there is now sugar contained in foods that you would not expect to have any sugar added. Most of the time, sweet tasting foods usually have sugar substitutes that taste like sugar but can have more damaging health effects than sugar itself.

- Sugar substitutes include such things as Aspartame, Saccharin, Splenda, High Fructose Corn Syrup, etc. Many of the packaged foods that so many people eat on a daily basis have at least some sugar added – even if the food doesn't register as sweet to your palate. A diet which is too high in sugars may lead to Candida (yeast) overgrowth, which can potentially lead to weight gain. The sugars you are ingesting feed the yeast, and the problems grow from there. Consider detoxing from much of the sugar you consume on a daily basis and you just may be amazed at the progress you can make.

As is so often the case when it comes to weight loss, it is best to think simply about the concept of detoxification. First we need to cleanse the body of the buildup of toxins that have accumulated already and then cleanse the cells that have been damaged from those toxins.

Second, to keep the body free from toxins, look for real foods which have been modified as little as possible on the way to your mouth. If you can gradually replace the toxic foods you eat with those which are natural and healthful, you are only going to move your health in a positive direction. The challenge of losing weight and regaining a healthy feeling can seem like a daunting one, but it really is all about making one good decision after another. Before long, if you pile up enough good decisions, you can radically change the way you eat and the way you live.

CHAPTER FOUR

ESSENTIAL VITAMINS AND MINERALS

Life is all about energy. It is hard to enjoy life when you are low on energy, and it can feel like the sky is the limit when your energy is overflowing. Despite its importance, it is hard to figure out exactly what energy is and where it comes from. For many people, there is a lack of understanding on this point which leads to poor decisions when it comes to things like diet and exercise.

The energy you feel on a daily basis is a direct result of the fuel you are putting into your body. You can think of this just like you would think about putting fuel into your car. If your vehicle runs on gasoline, and you put quality gas into the tank, you will expect to get good performance. However, if you put water in the tank instead, the car is quickly going to come to a stop. It's not quite that simple with your body, but the idea is the same. Give your body plenty of good fuel and it is going to have all the energy you need to get through the day. Give your body the wrong kind of fuel, or not enough fuel, and you are sure to 'hit the wall' at some point.

In addition to maintaining a healthy weight to avoid negative health conditions and to look your best, you will also want to focus on this point simply because it will allow you to have more energy. With more energy, you should immediately begin to enjoy life more on a day to day basis. If you have been obese for many years, you may be surprised to find how much you can get done in a single day now that you have plenty of energy once again.

There is a direct connection between carrying too much weight and having a lack of energy. When you are overweight, your body has to work harder to do everything, all day long. From simply getting up out of a chair to walking across a parking lot, every task you take on is harder. By the end of the day, these tasks add up and you wind up feeling quite fatigued. In fact, for those people who are extremely overweight, it won't even take until the end of the day. Fatigue can set in by lunch time, and it may not let go until the next morning.

Of course, there is another thing to think about with regard to obesity and fatigue. When you are overweight, it is very likely that you are eating a diet which is less-than-ideal. That means plenty of processed foods, a lot of sugar, and very little nutrition. These are the foods that have caused you to become overweight in the first place, and they are also part of the reason that you don't have very much energy. Your body is looking for specific vitamins and minerals to use as fuel during your day, but it might not find those to be available when you eat a bad diet. Once all of the refined sugar is used up, you will likely feel a 'crash' and you will have very little energy left.

To correct this problem, it should go without saying that you need to correct your diet. By eating more of the good stuff – fresh fruits and veggies, whole grains, nuts, etc. – you can provide your body with exactly what it is looking for when fuel is necessary. All of the right vitamins and minerals will be in abundant supply and you should be able to move your weight in the right direction as well.

A big step toward your ultimate destination is making sure to provide your body with the essential vitamins and minerals it needs. Consuming these in liquid form can be advantageous thanks to the ease with which the body can absorb them; but simply getting vitamins and minerals into your body in any safe manner is helpful in a variety of ways.

- Vitamins and minerals can boost your immune system

- They can help to heal wounds and make bones stronger
- Also can help release energy from food
- Improved digestion and metabolism
- Benefits your heart health

For those who are significantly overweight, one of the biggest problems is just getting started on the journey to a healthy physical condition. After all, if you need to lose 100 pounds or more, that ultimate goal can feel like it is a lifetime away. Fortunately, on the topic of energy, you won't have to wait all that long in order to see some very real benefits. If you make changes to the way you eat, and you drop even a few pounds in the early going, it is likely that you will feel that you have more energy throughout the day. And, as you start to enjoy those energetic feelings, you will only be more and more motivated to keep up with your newfound diet and exercise habits. This is a process that can build on itself, with each small victory pushing you forward to work even harder.

In many ways, the potential to regain lost energy is one of the most exciting things about losing weight and eating healthier foods. Sure, it might be nice to fit into some pants that have long been shoved to the back of your closet, but appearance concerns should be secondary to how you feel each day. With more energy available, a whole new world may open up. You might perform better at work, you may feel up to engaging in new hobbies, and you should have more energy to play with your kids. Whatever the reason for wanting more energy, it is never too late to make changes that will allow you to feel your best day after day.

ACIDITY/ ALKALIZATION

In this section, we are going to talk about something that can be a little intimidating to many people – at least at first. You might not understand the importance of your body's pH at the moment, but it should soon become clear that this is an important topic related to your health.

First, let's go through a quick review of pH, in case you have forgotten from your high school science classes. pH is a measure of hydrogen ion concentration. pH can be measured in many areas, and in this case, we are talking about the pH in your body. The pH scale runs from 1 up to 14, with anything below 7 considered acidic, and anything over 7 considered alkaline. The foods we eat also have their own pH level, meaning you can manipulate the pH in your body – at least to some degree – by picking and choosing the right kinds of foods.

It is thought that the ideal place to land on this scale is close to neutral, just on the alkaline side of the middle. There are a variety of negative health outcomes that may at least be partially related to acidity in the body, including digestive disorders, circulatory system problems, immune system issues, and more. By eating more foods that land on the alkaline side of the scale, you should be able to move your pH in the right direction, and potentially steer clear of some of these undesirable health issues.

An acidic environment is considered the perfect setting for illness and disease to thrive in. Previously, the acid-alkaline diet was thought to be some crazy, vegan hippie myth. But even Dr. Otto Warburg, who dedicated his life to researching cancer cells, won a Nobel Prize for proving that cancer cells cannot survive in an alkaline environment.

One of the primary factors that influence our blood's pH are the kinds of foods we eat.

All foods can be categorized as acidic, alkaline, or neutral. A food's pH isn't measured by its physical properties, but by the residue that's left in the body once the food has been metabolized.

The Problem with Being Too Acidic

We've briefly touched on one of the most detrimental effects of an acidic internal environment, which is the encouragement of disease – specifically cancer.

But being too acidic can come with other symptoms that occur far before a serious illness results. In fact, being too acidic can result in muscle wasting and reduced bone density. This is partially due to the fact that many acidic foods are low in nutrients that promote musculoskeletal health, such as potassium and calcium.

To get slightly more scientific in terms of bone health, an acidic environment has been shown to encourage the activity of osteoclast cells. Osteoclasts are cells that break down bone. In contrast, an alkaline environment has been shown to encourage the activity of osteoblasts, which are the cells that help build bone.

In addition to the long-term conditions that can result from being too acidic, there are short-term symptoms that may also suggest your body is more on the acidic end of the pH scale.

These symptoms include:

- Low energy
- Exhaustion
- Acne
- Brain fog or confusion
- Anxiety and depression
- Frequent headaches
- Frequent colds
- Joint pain
- Muscle weakness
- Digestive issues such as bloating, constipation and weight gain

Now, the body contains natural compounds such as bicarbonate that act as buffers to neutralize blood acidity. These buffers help prevent extreme drops in blood pH. This is an important defense not only against acidifying foods, but also against other factors that promote acidity in the body, such as chronic stress.

Strenuous exercise can also promote blood acidity because it encourages the release of lactic acid from the muscle tissue.

While your body has a natural defense system against having an acidic blood pH, it is possible for these buffers to get worn out over time – especially if several factors are present that negatively impact your pH, such as stress and a highly acidic diet. For this reason, it's important to support your body by including alkaline foods in your diet whenever possible.

This isn't to say you must go raw vegan and eat only alkalizing fruits and vegetables for the rest of your life.

While it's rare, it's still possible for the blood to become too alkaline. But since the modern diet is typically higher in acidifying foods, including alkalizing foods into your diet each day will help neutralize your blood pH and improve your health in numerous ways.

So, what kinds of foods should you be eating in order to go in the alkaline direction? Well, it should be no surprise whatsoever to find that the foods that come in on the alkaline side are those that you already know to be good for your body. That's right, those very same fruits and vegetables that we have been talking about throughout this book so far are going to help you in this regard, as well. And, the foods that you probably already know to avoid are ones that you should avoid for pH reasons, too.

The list below includes some of the many foods that are desirable from an alkalinity perspective.

- Apples, bananas, strawberries, grapefruit, peaches, pineapple
- Avocadoes, lettuce, celery, sweet potatoes, green beans, spinach, broccoli
- Onions, mushrooms, wild rice, olives, asparagus, kale

In the following list, we have included some of the items that come in on the acidic side of the scale. You probably aren't going to be very surprised by the entries below, but we needed to highlight them just to prove the point.

- Pastries, chocolate, sweetened fruit juice, cocoa, popcorn
- Beer, wine
- Pasta, buttermilk, cheese, beef

- Ultra-processed foods, such as frozen dinners, store-bought cakes, etc.
- Caffeinated drinks
- Processed cereals
- Artificial sweeteners
- Peanuts
- Rice
- Bread
- Wheat products
- Cold cut meats

And so it goes. Maintaining regular pH levels is critical to health. Eating too many acidic foods may alter hormone levels, contribute to chronic pain and even weaken the bones. It can also lower the pH of your urine, which may result in the development of certain types of kidney stones. There are also certain types of acidic food that can cause the triggering of acid reflux symptoms.

As you should understand by this point in the book, there are few real surprises when it comes to nutrition. Often, you need nothing more than your gut instinct to tell you whether or not a particular food is a healthy choice. While it is incredibly important to make sure your body is getting all of the vitamins and minerals it needs, and while you should be concerned about your pH, you don't have to use any complicated formulas to find the right food. Fresh foods, mostly fruits and vegetables, will take you nearly all the way to an ideal diet.

It is important when getting into topics like alkalization to not become overwhelmed by the science on the potential complexity of it all. As an individual who needs to lose weight and get your health back on track, your jobs are really quite simple in the end. You need to eat healthy foods, you need to eat a healthy amount of food, and you need to live a more active lifestyle. That's it. Yes, pH is important. But as we've demonstrated above, eating foods which are generally considered to be healthful will automatically take you in the right direction from a pH perspective.

If you are interested in the idea of alkalizing the body, one option is to drink alkaline water. This is a product which is readily available today in a number of locations. If you are one of the many people who regularly consume acidic products like coffee and sodas, drinking alkaline water may be able to balance things out and help you lose weight over the long run. Of course, your personal experience will depend on a number of factors.

CHAPTER SIX

LOW OR IMBALANCED HORMONES

Some things in life get easier as we age. For example, most people make more money as they get older and gain experience, so they are more able to pay their bills month after month. Also, we tend to get wiser and more patient as we age, so the things that may have bothered you during your youth will just roll off your back in your later years. In many ways, it is a good thing to have plenty of years in your rearview mirror.

When it comes to the hormones in your body, however, it is hard to see age as an advantage. As your body ages, there will likely be changes taking place in your systems which result in your hormones making less of an impact on the way your body operates. In some cases, it is that your hormone production has decreased, while in other cases it is simply that your tissues are not as responsive to the hormones that control them. Whatever the case, most people notice hormonal changes as they age.

Why Hormones Matter.

The hormones in your body are responsible for an incredible amount of what takes place inside you on a day to day basis. While they are rarely thought of as you go about your day, they are working in the background, keeping many of your systems in order. You have a number of glands in your body which are responsible for producing hormones including the hypothalamus, the thyroid, the pituitary and many others.

For your body to function properly, it is important to have various hormones being produced at proper levels. Most people are aware of estrogen and testosterone being the prevalent sex hormones in women and men, respectively. There are, however, other lesser known hormones that can contribute to weight gain if they are low or out of balance.

Let's first take a look at these and how they can contribute to weight gain. First is melatonin, which is a hormone that is associated with your ability to sleep, and as such it increases after dark. When your body is stressed and you have too much on your mind keeping you awake at night, you can be assured that your melatonin levels are out of balance. The correlation between sleep and weight gain occurs for a handful of reasons. When you don't get enough sleep and need more energy, you may find yourself reaching for excess amounts of food to provide the necessary fuel. Research shows that the less sleep you get, the more likely you are to store fat and take in more calories. When you are tired, you tend to reach for food or caffeine to keep you going. Because of this, adequate sleep (at least seven and a half hours) is important to maintain weight levels. When your endocrine system is working properly to produce and distribute your hormones successfully, your body can function as it is meant to in a variety of key ways. If there is a problem with your sleep and melatonin levels, you are likely to notice the side effects of that issue.

Another important hormone that can get out of balance is cortisol, which is the body's main stress hormone. It's released whenever your body senses it needs to enter 'high-alert mode' - whether you're facing a major work deadline, fighting with your significant other, or even just hammering away in the gym. Cortisol raises blood pressure and blood sugar to power your muscles and causes your body to go into a fight-or-flight mode. Cortisol basically suppresses all body processes (like your immune response, digestion, and reproductive function) that would be nonessential in a true flight-or-fight situation. While cortisol may help your body handle some sort of threat or stress in the short-term, it becomes an issue if it's chronically elevated. Cortisol becomes poison, causing you to store belly fat, deplete your 'happy' brain chemicals like serotonin and lose sleep. These issues can snowball and lead to headaches, anxiety, depression, and digestive problems long-term. Elevated cortisol levels are also linked to food addiction and sugar cravings, and leave you more likely to reach for processed, unhealthy foods. The best way to support healthy cortisol function is to evaluate and manage the stress in your life. Practicing things like yoga, meditation, getting a massage, chiropractic adjustments, acupuncture, or seeing a counseling professional to help get symptoms under control will help control cortisol and your weight.

The next important hormone is insulin, which is a hormone made in the pancreas that allows your body to use glucose (a.k.a. sugar) for energy. When you eat or drink something that contains sugar, your body releases insulin to clear that sugar from your blood and shuttle it to your tissues (like muscles) for use.

When your cells become numb to insulin, you develop insulin resistance and instead of shuttling glucose from your blood into your cells, your liver converts that sugar into stored fat. The condition is often marked by intense sugar cravings and weight gain and experts believe excess weight and inactivity are both major factors in causing it. Losing weight and exercising is vitally important when your body is resistant to insulin because long term insulin resistance can lead to diabetes which can cause damage to your eyes, kidneys, and nerves (diabetic neuropathy). It can also cause heart disease, stroke and even the need to remove a limb.

If insulin is the fat storage hormone then glucagon is the fat burning hormone. Glucagon's job is to signal the fat cells to release free fatty acids (a process called lipolysis) so that the body can release the stored fat to be used as fuel. Numerous research studies illustrate the effects of insulin and glucagon being opposing hormones. Simply put, insulin promotes fat storage and it keeps you fat by blocking access to your fat reserves. Glucagon is essential for breaking down body fat and burning it for energy.

If you want to convert your body to a perpetual fat-burning state, it is essential that you keep your insulin and blood sugar levels low. That's because burning sugar always takes precedence over burning fat. The more carbohydrates in your diet, the higher your blood sugar and insulin levels will be. And in the end, being a "sugar burner" means you'll end up being a "fat accumulator". But that's not the worst of it because once you get on the sugar-burning track, you've started a vicious cycle that's hard to stop.

Since your body is accustomed to burning sugar for energy, as soon as it is shuttled out of the bloodstream (courtesy of insulin), your body will start begging for it again. As your blood sugar rises and subsequently crashes, you will become edgy, depressed and fatigued until those cravings are fed. When you feed those cravings with more carb-rich food, the cycle continues.

As I mentioned earlier, the production of insulin and glucagon are like a see-saw. So the first thing you need to do to stimulate the production of glucagon is to reduce total carbohydrates (grains, alcohol, sugar and starches) in your diet and be sure those you choose are low glycemic. But there's another important step to crank up your body's production of glucagon: Eat a protein-rich diet!

Protein directly stimulates the production of glucagon and sends the signal to your body that the "hunting is good" and it is safe to shed excess fat. Protein also promotes a long-lasting feeling of fullness, helping you to stay satisfied on a diet of fewer calories.

Here are the high quality protein sources you should choose from and include at every meal and snack:

- Grass-fed beef and lamb
- Wild seafood (sardines, mackerel, wild salmon, etc)
- Pastured poultry
- Game meats (bison, elk, rabbit, etc)
- Pastured eggs
- Grass-fed whey protein

The plan for shedding fat and keeping it off forever is very simple and requires no deprivation.

The key is to consume plenty of protein and healthy fats. And be sure that the carbs you choose are low glycemic and high in fiber. By eating this way, your hormonal state will shift from that of a "sugar burner" to a "fat burner."

You will soon discover that you feel more satisfied on less food. Your between-meal cravings will subside. And best of all, your metabolism will fire on all cylinders, locking your body into a perpetual fat-burning state.

Not many people talk about leptin but this is another important hormone because it is another big influencer on hunger and satiety. It is known as your appetite suppressant hormone. Under normal conditions, leptin signals your brain to stop eating once you've had enough to eat. Leptin is released from your fat cells, so research suggests that adequate leptin signals to our body that we have enough fat and aren't starving, and consequently don't need to take in tons of calories.

However, when leptin levels (and body fat) keep rising, your receptors stop functioning properly and you never quite get the leptin cue that you're satisfied, which annoyingly leaves you feeling hungry. Known as leptin resistance, this predicament leaves you more likely to continue to snack on unhealthy foods and can cause weight gain to snowball. This has been identified in research as leptin resistance and is a major player in obesity.

So to recap, extra abdominal belly fat can indicate that one or more of the following hormonal imbalances exists: high estrogen, low testosterone, low DHEA (a hormone of the adrenal glands), low glucagon,high insulin, high leptin and high cortisol.

Abdominal fat also sets a risky stage for aging, increasing the risk of heart disease and diabetes. A program to get rid of this stubborn fat must include proper diet, exercise, sleep and, of course, motivation. All of these components work well to instill a healthy balance that allows fat loss to occur.

It is important to understand how hormones can affect weight gain, especially in older people. To highlight this concept, let's look at what can happen to a middle-age woman after going through the process of menopause. It is extremely common for women to gain weight after menopause, and it seems that the hormone estrogen is at least partly to blame for this phenomenon.

There have been studies in animals to indicate that the body uses estrogen in part to control weight. When the estrogen level in women drops after menopause, it is possible that the metabolic rate will drop as well. That means that without making any dietary or exercise changes, a woman may gain a relatively significant amount of weight. It might not be fair that you could wind up gaining weight simply by aging and having lower hormone levels, but you'll have to deal with it just the same.

Some Options

For women who have gained weight as a side effect of menopause, it isn't necessary to just sit back and accept that outcome. There are steps that can be taken to move your weight back into a healthier range. Of course, maintaining a healthy weight is always important for your overall health, so this is not something that is just about how you look.

One possible solution is the use of a hormone cream, like those that deliver progesterone to the body. Progesterone is another hormone which can be affected by menopause, so using a cream is a possible way to re-balance this important hormone. Also, a cream which helps to elevate DHEA may be able to assist in the increase of your metabolic rate. Of course, as is always the case, you want to check with your doctor before using a hormone cream or any other kind of treatment.

As another option, it may be helpful to simply review your diet and exercise plan both during and after menopause. If your body's needs are changing as you age, it is important to respond to those changes with the right adjustments. It is certainly possible for older people to stay at a healthy weight, so making wise choices with regard to diet and exercise could be all that is necessary to get your weight back on track.

CHAPTER SEVEN

FUEL

Earlier in this book, we touched on the topic of viewing your food as fuel. We compared eating food on a daily basis to putting fuel in your car. The gasoline you put into your vehicle is going to be used to propel the car down the road. Just the same, the food you put into your body is going to help keep your body moving all day long. No matter what you happen to be doing on a given day, the food you consume is going to play a large role in your productivity, in addition to helping determine how you feel.

In the modern world, we tend to think about food more as an opportunity for pleasure than anything else. Rather than picking foods based on what they can do for your body and your health, most people pick food based on what tastes good in the moment. This phenomenon can help explain the popularity of fast food, which is bad for your health by nearly every measure. If you were picking food based on its ability to fuel your body's needs, you would never go anywhere near a fast food restaurant. When picking based only on your immediate urges, however, it is easy to pull into the drive-thru for a cheap burger and fries.

Not only will fast food be bad for your health over the long term, it will likely make you feel poorly in just a matter of hours. Do you feel full of energy after your body has had time to digest a fast food meal? Probably not.

More likely, you will feel sluggish, lethargic, and tired. You might even have a stomach ache. By prioritizing your short-term desire for something salty and greasy, you have negatively impacted your health for both the short- and long-term. Needless to say, it would be in your best interest to make better decisions.

It's Not All About Fast Food

When talking about weight loss, fast food is an easy target. Of course, hearing that fast food is not good for your health probably isn't breaking news. What you may not know is there are just as many troublesome foods available at the grocery store as are available at the local fast food joint. Most people tend to think of the grocery store as a way to eat healthier – and it can certainly be that – but nothing is guaranteed until you fill up your basket with the right items. If you don't know what to buy, you can do just as much damage to your health in the grocery store as anywhere else you might acquire food.

The big enemy in the modern mega-mart is processed food. More and more people are becoming aware of the negative impact that processed foods can have on your health, but this is a message that needs to keep expanding. Hopefully, in the not too distant future, the average consumer will put processed foods in the same category as fast food in terms of things that are to be avoided for the benefit of your health.

So, what's so wrong about picking out processed food items in the grocery store? Let's take a look at a few of the potential problems with these types of foods.

- **Excess Sugar** - In the right form, there isn't anything wrong with consuming a modest amount of sugar. When you eat a piece of fruit, for example, you will be consuming natural sugar, along with things like fiber, vitamins, minerals, etc. And, of course, eating a piece of fruit is a healthy dietary option. However, when you obtain sugar through processed foods, it is likely to come in much too high of a quantity, and in the wrong form. Many processed foods are sweetened with high fructose corn syrup, which is able to deliver a huge dose of sugar to your body in a relatively small package. By obtaining your sugar from natural sources, you will get it in smaller doses, and you may be able to avoid the negative health effects of consuming large quantities of processed sugar. It is important to note that you need to be careful when shopping, as even foods that don't taste sweet can be packed with high fructose corn syrup. Take a quick look at the label to determine what is in any processed food that you may purchase.

- **Salt Overload** - Not only will you find excessive amounts of sugar in many processed foods, you are also likely to come across significant amounts of sodium. Again, this is a point you should be checking carefully on the label of all packaged foods. Since salt is an excellent way to preserve food, packaged items are often made salty as a way to keep them shelf stable. Of course, the salty nature of the food also appeals to your taste buds, which the food company hopes will keep you coming back for more. Just as was the case with sugar, it is not that salt is inherently bad for you. In fact, your body requires salt. Unfortunately, it is the dose which is the issue. Too much salt can lead to a number of negative health outcomes, including the potential for things like high blood pressure, heart attack, and stroke. Many people wind up consuming too much salt through processed foods, and they never even know that it's happening. Since they aren't actually shaking the salt onto their food themselves, it is easy to forget that it is lurking 'behind the scenes'. When you do need to add salt to your foods, consider Himalayan pink salt as an option. A variety of minerals are present in this type of salt, so it can serve a purpose other than just improving the taste of your food.

- **Collection of Chemicals** - If you pull a packaged food out of your pantry, you are likely to find an incredibly long list of ingredients. And, among those ingredients, are likely to be a number of words that you can't even pronounce. Most likely, these are chemicals which have been added to your food in order to preserve, add color, change the texture, or make some other alteration. Are these chemicals dangerous? Well, that depends on who you believe. What is pretty clear, however, is that they are not adding nutritional value to your diet. If you do need to buy processed food from time to time, it is a good rule of thumb to look for short ingredient lists, and try to find products with ingredients that you recognize. The more real food that is actually present in your diet, the better. By opting for real food, you may be able to avoid consuming too much of certain types of oils, such as vegetable oil, palm oil and partially hydrogenated oils. If you take in too much vegetable oil or other similar oils, you may be getting far too much Omega-6 fatty acid, which may lead to a variety of negative outcomes.

- **Calorie rich, nutrient poor** - One of the worst things you can say about any type of food is that it is high in calories and low in nutrition. These kinds of foods aren't going to provide your body much in the way of fuel, but they will pack your diet with calories. Ideally, you would like your food to be the opposite. Healthy foods – things like fruits and vegetables – tend to have a lot of nutrients and relatively few calories. Eating these foods tends to be the most effective and efficient way to fuel your body.

In the battle against obesity, processed and packaged foods should be seen as just as big of an enemy as fast food. With that said, not all packaged foods in the grocery store are bad choices. In recent years, some companies have made a concerted effort to create healthier options for shoppers who want to make good choices. This is a great development, as there certainly is something to be said for the convenience of processed food.

Your job, of course, is to sort out the good from the bad each time you step foot in the grocery store. To start with, always read labels carefully on processed foods before you buy them. If you see too many things that you can't pronounce, or you find high levels of things like salt and high fructose corn syrup, it will be better to take a pass. Most likely, the packaged foods worth eating are going to be sold in the health foods section of your grocery store, but even foods on those aisles are no guarantee of nutrition. Always read labels, and do your best to prioritize fresh foods over packaged options whenever possible.

How Does Your Body Use Food as Fuel?

So much of what your body does on a daily basis goes on behind the scenes. You don't have to think about it – and you may not even understand it. For instance, how does your body take the food you eat and convert it into fuel that you can use to get through the day? While that topic is far too complex for the scope of this book, we will provide a basic overview below so you can become familiar with the general concept.

When thinking about the way your body uses food as fuel, you can break down the foods you eat into three major categories – carbohydrates, fats, and proteins. To start, we will look at carbs, as they are the major source of energy within your body. When you consume carbohydrates like sugars or starches, those are quickly broken down into glucose, and your body can then use the glucose to supply you with the energy you need to complete the task at hand.

If you think of fat only in a negative way with regard to your diet, you will need to rethink once you learn that fat is actually an important source of energy. Your body stores fat as an energy reserve, and it is a powerful reserve at that. Fat is a more concentrated source of energy than carbohydrates, which is why healthy fats can be considered an important part of well-rounded diet. If you don't have any fats available, you will quickly run out of energy once your available glucose has been used up.

What kinds of fats are 'good' fats? Generally speaking, unsaturated fats are considered to be good fats, in that they can provide your body with some important benefits. Of course, everything in the diet realm needs to be managed in moderation, so good fats are only good when they are consumed in reasonable quantities. There are plenty of sources of good fats available, but some of the most popular options include olives, peanut oil, avocados, nuts, seeds, fish oil, and more.

Finally, we arrive at protein. If you've done much reading on nutrition topics, or if you've ever visited a health food store, you might get the impression that you need to pack your body with loads and loads of protein in order to be healthy. That simply isn't the case. While protein is essential to be sure, your body really isn't going to turn to protein for energy in most cases.

It is true that your body can turn to protein for energy when other reserves are depleted, but you'll do well to avoid these situations. You would rather have your available protein go to work doing things like building and repairing body tissues. When your protein is used for energy purposes, it can lead to the breakdown of lean muscle mass. Make no mistake – protein is an important part of a healthy diet, but it isn't a major source of energy, at least when compared to carbohydrates and fat.

A Slow, Even Burn

As you go through your day, you should be gradually supplying your body with fuel that can be used to keep you feeling your best. Unless you are taking part in a particularly taxing form of exercise – which will require its own plan for fueling – you will simply need to make sure none of your energy reserves run out completely. When you do run out of energy, specifically in the form of glucose, there are some very noticeable side effects.

For example, have you ever found yourself at work late in the afternoon, feeling unable to focus on the task at hand? You know you have work to do, you are willing to do it, but you just can't manage to focus your brain on the job in front of you. When these feelings set in, there is a good chance they are related to your energy levels. If you had a big lunch full of sugars and fats, your body had plenty of energy available for a couple hours after that meal. The 'crash', however, is soon to follow. When your glucose level drops, your energy and ability to focus will go with it. In this way, failing to manage your diet properly can have a very real effect on your ability to perform well on the job.

Although it is modern custom for people to eat three large meals in the form of breakfast, lunch, and dinner, there is plenty of reason to believe it would be better to simply eat fewer meals and focus more on longer periods of fasting. Intermittent fasting is one of the best ways for the body to utilize stored fats. It may take some time to get used to going longer between meals, but you can eventually retrain your brain with regard to when you feel like you need to eat.

Also, there is the option of taking on a ketogenic (fat burning) diet in order to maintain a fat burning state within your body. While an entire other book could be dedicated to the ketogenic diet, the basic idea is that this is a low carb diet which pushes the body into ketosis. This can result in the body using fat as an energy source, rather than glucose. A keto diet is not likely to be the best bet for everyone, but it is something to consider as you are making a plan to move forward.

As many people are looking for the perfect food intake plan for their body, most Americans continue to struggle with being overfed but undernourished. Most people are challenged with consuming food for pleasure instead of consuming for proper fuel. As a baby step toward a better fueling plan, try simply eating a little less at each meal and then regain those calories by eating more healthy snacks between meals. This is going to be an adjustment at first, but you may soon find that you feel better throughout the day – especially in the late afternoon, which is a common time for people to 'run out of steam'. Of course, it is crucial that those snacks you add are healthy ones, as choosing unhealthy snacks is not going to do you any good. Plan out your fueling strategy for each day ahead of time and always have the right foods on hand to keep yourself going.

CHAPTER EIGHT

EXERCISE

Up to this point, we have talked exclusively about the diet portion of weight loss. What you put into your body on a daily basis has a huge impact on your weight, and your overall health, so that topic needed to be covered extensively. However, it is still only one piece of the puzzle, and now it is time to turn to another key piece – exercise. If you aren't the type to be excited at the thought of a long day of physical activity, don't worry. You don't necessarily have to be an endurance athlete to get the kind of exercise required to lower your body weight over time.

Before we get started in this chapter, it is important to note that you should always have the approval of a doctor before you get started on any exercise regimen. You need to be sure that your health will support the kinds of activities you plan to take on, so always be cautious and seek medical approval before moving into the exercise part of the process.

Some Basic Math

If you are going to lose weight, you need to operate at a calorie deficit day after day. That simply means that you need to make sure your body is burning more calories than you are taking in throughout the day. Some people attempt to tackle this hurdle by simply not eating very much food, while also avoiding exercise. It is possible for this to work, but there are a couple of major problems. For one thing, eating very few calories during the day will put you at risk of missing out on important nutrients. Unless you are eating a perfectly designed diet plan created for you by a nutritionist, you may miss out on things you need when your calories are severely restricted.

Another issue here is simply feeling hungry throughout the day. You might be able to 'suck it up' for a while and deal with your hunger, but it is going to get the best of you at some point. In the meantime, you'll probably be irritable, frustrated, and generally unpleasant. When people seem like they are struggling with weight loss, it is often because they are trying to lose weight simply by slashing their caloric intake while making no other changes.

Unfortunately, this style of weight loss winds up being a failure for most people. To give yourself a better chance of success, it would be wise to consider adding exercise to your routine. Basically, exercise is going to give you a chance to change the math with regard to calories in and calories out. During exercise, your body is going to burn more calories that it would use up if you were just sitting in a chair. That means you'll be able to afford to eat more calories during the day while still winding up with a calorie deficit. It will be easier to get all of the necessary nutrients, because you'll be eating more calories, and you might not have to feel hungry as often. Even modest exercise can help you burn some additional calories, and that bit of additional burn just might make the difference when you step on the scale.

Picking the Right Options

For many people, one of the biggest challenges of adding exercise to a weight loss plan is simply finding the right type of exercise. There are tons of options available today for exercise, so you can feel free to pick something that suits you nicely. As you think about how you are going to get your exercise moving forward, keep the following points in mind.

- Where will you exercise? This is one of the first topics to consider. Are you going to exercise at home/outside, or are you going to join a gym? There are pros and cons to each option. When you choose to join a gym, the two drawbacks are the monthly cost and the time it takes to travel to the gym. On the plus side, you will have access to a variety of machines, you will be able to work out indoors when the weather is bad, and you might find it motivating to be around other people who are working toward their fitness goals. For those who stay at home, there is no monthly cost (although you may need to buy some equipment upfront), and you are always just steps away from starting a workout. Going for a walk or run outside is enjoyable for many people, and you won't have to worry about being self-conscious as you might if you visit a gym. Of course, a home gym is not going to have the same kind of equipment as a commercial gym, there won't be anyone else around to motivate you, and you won't have access to professional trainers. In the end, there is no right or wrong decision on this point. Think about your own situation, and your own personality, to decide which option is best.

- What kind of exercise? You might need to experiment a bit here before you land on something that works for you. The most basic forms of exercise are walking and running, as you don't need equipment other than comfortable shoes and appropriate apparel. If those don't seem like a good fit, you can try biking, swimming, elliptical machines, fitness classes, etc. One key to keep in mind on this point is any injuries or physical limitations that you need to consider. For example, running is fantastic exercise from a fitness stand point, as you will burn a significant number of calories in a relatively short period of time. However, it can be hard for some people to stay healthy when running consistently, with various foot, ankle, or leg injuries popping up over time. The best exercise is the exercise that allows you to burn calories while staying healthy over the long run. After all, a challenging workout doesn't do you much good if it puts you out of commission for a couple weeks while you recover. If you haven't done much exercise in recent years, or if you have never done much exercise in your life, it is best to start with low intensity options and work your way up gradually.

- Alone, or in a group? Some people love to work out alone. They enjoy the quiet time as they focus on improving their body and clearing their mind at the same time. You might find that your exercise routine becomes an enjoyable opportunity to slow down the busy pace of your life for a bit. On the other hand, solo exercise is simply boring for other people. These people don't like the feeling of being alone with their thoughts, and would rather workout in a group. If that sounds more like you, it is relatively easy to find other people to share in your newfound workout habit. You might be able to join fitness classes at a gym, join a local running group, or take part in a club that focuses on whatever you have chosen as your preferred type of exercise.

Even when you have decided on the type of exercise that you will use as your main option, it is still a good idea to mix it up from time to time. There really isn't such thing as a 'perfect' activity which will address your entire body, so try to find a variety of ways to get your exercise as the weeks and months go by. For example, if you have decided to jog/run for most of your exercise, you might wind up doing that three or four times per week. On the other days, you could go for a bike ride, attend a yoga class, or workout with a trainer at your local gym. Whatever it is, mixing up your routine will usually mean nothing but good things for your overall fitness.

Finding the Sweet Spot

Once you start to get excited about losing weight, it is easy to get carried away with the exercise piece of the puzzle. This is not all bad, of course, as exercise is great for your overall health, and it is a powerful tool when trying to lose weight. Unfortunately, it is possible to get a bit carried away at first, and you might wind up paying for it in the end. You need to find the 'sweet spot' for exercise in terms of how often you will work out, and how intense those workouts will be.

If you exercise too much right from the start, or if you work out too hard, there are a number of negative consequences which could be waiting. Those include the following –

- Injury. This is the most obvious potential problem which could stem from exercising too much early in your weight loss journey. If you injure yourself early on, you will have to back off of your exercise in order to recover. This will be frustrating, and it might set you back for quite some time. While it is hard to be patient in this situation, gradually ramping up your exercise is the right way to go. If you take it easy at the start and slowly increase the duration and intensity of your workouts as you go, it is more likely that you'll be able to stay healthy. Even a relatively minor injury – like some mild tendonitis – can prevent you from exercising properly, so never take the threat of injury for granted.

- Burn out. This point doesn't have to do with physical injury, but rather mental fatigue. If you jump right into an aggressive workout plan, exercising nearly every day of the week, you might quickly get tired of your new routine. Too much of anything can be hard to maintain, and that is certainly true of exercise. Ideally, you would like to get to a point where you can genuinely enjoy your exercise each day. If you look forward to it, you will be more likely to stick with it over time. To avoid burning out early on, hold yourself back and limit how many exercise sessions you complete each week. In time, you will get more and more comfortable with your various workouts, and you should be able to increase the frequency of your workouts without much risk of getting burned out. Also, variety is a good way to stave off boredom, so make sure to mix up your workouts if you feel burnout coming on.

- Putting too much pressure on your diet. Most people decide to make dietary changes at the same time they are getting started with a new exercise plan, which can be tough. Your body is going to be adjusting to some new foods, and probably fewer calories throughout the course of the day. At the same time, your body might need to adjust to a new exercise routine, with the additional calorie burn and some sore muscles as well. If you take all this on at the same time, and you push yourself hard during the workouts, it is likely that you will quickly find yourself lacking for energy. While your improved diet is still new, maintain a modest exercise regimen and work on building it up as your body continues to adjust.

The lesson here is simple – don't go all in on exercise right from the start. Instead, think about finding a sweet spot which is both effective and sustainable. As you gain experience with regular workouts, you will start to get familiar with how they impact your body, and you'll learn what you can handle without too much trouble. Constantly monitor the way you feel and adjust your workout plans as necessary moving forward.

Is Walking Really Exercise?

For those who are significantly overweight, it can be quite the challenge to get started with a regular habit of exercise. Excess weight makes some types of exercise, such as running or bike riding, rather difficult at first. That isn't to say you can't work your way into those kinds of exercise in time, but they might not be a good fit at the start. So, is it okay to start out by using nothing but walking as your form of exercise?

Of course – there is nothing wrong with using walking as your exercise of choice. In fact, it is easy to argue that walking is the best way of all to get started working toward your health goals. Walking is low-impact, meaning you are less likely to injure your muscles or joints in the process. And, walking is free, unless you choose to join a gym to do your walking on a treadmill. Given good weather, you can fit in a walk outside your home or near your office anytime you have a few minutes available. You don't need any specialized equipment beyond what you probably already own, and you don't need anyone to teach you how to do it. When you look at it this way, it is easy to see just how appealing it can be to use walking as a starting point in your fitness journey.

With all of that said, there is a good chance that you are going to 'outgrow' walking at some point along the way. In other words, as you begin to lose weight and improve your fitness, you'll probably reach a point where simply walking for exercise isn't taxing your body enough to achieve any notable results. When you do get to that point, you may need to start thinking about other options to increase the intensity of your exercise. There is no rush to get to this point, however. A habit of walking for exercise is much better than no exercise at all, so be proud of yourself for taking this first step, and look forward to even bigger steps to come.

Not a Free Pass

One of the main lessons we hope to pass along through this book is the fact that diet and exercise need to work together if you are going to reach your weight loss goals. The strategy you use should be a complimentary one, with each side of the equation holding up its end of the bargain. It is with that in mind that we need to point out the fact that simply exercising regularly is not a free pass to eat whatever you want.

Simply put, you can't exercise enough to make up for a bad diet and/or lifestyle. For example, it takes a significant amount of time and energy to burn a few hundred calories while exercising. However, it only takes a few minutes to eat a calorie rich food which can more than replace all of the calories you managed to burn through your hard work. It would be a shame to waste all of the great work you did during your exercise session just because you decided to eat a couple of donuts (or some other calorie rich, nutrient poor food).

You are only going to have long-term success with your weight loss plan when you are able to match up your diet and exercise nicely. Sure, getting regular exercise might allow you to eat a little more food while still losing weight, but those need to be the right kinds of foods. They should be healthy, nutrient rich foods which deliver you many different vitamins and minerals. To keep yourself in check, always review the caloric intake of any food you are thinking about adding to your diet, and compare those calories to what you have burned during your workout. If you are going to consume a quick snack which has as many calories as your full workout, it might be wise to look for another snack option.

In the end, even though you may find the perfect food intake plan and have the perfect exercise routine, you may still find yourself having difficulty getting to your ideal weight. If that's the case, then referring back to the I.D.E.A.L. factors that we originally highlighted and seeing which ones you may be missing out on will most likely get you to your goal. You see, it's not just a matter of having the perfect food plan or exercise plan; it's about getting your body to function at its optimum potential to obtain the optimum results you're looking for.

CHAPTER NINE

MOTIVATION

For many people, this chapter is going to be the most important in the whole book. It is all well and good to understand what you need to do from a diet and exercise perspective, but how do you get it done? How do you stay motivated when you have so many other things to do in so many other parts of your life? To be sure, motivation can be hard to come by when you are trying to bring your body weight down into a healthy range.

An Individual Battle

One of the hardest things about staying motivated is the things that motivate you are going to be personal in nature. Your motivating factors might not mean anything to another person, while what motivates someone else might not do anything for you. In the end, the key to staying motivated over the long term is finding those things that really drive you to be your best. Only you can know what those are, but we'll do our best to help you uncover them.

Review the list below as a way to generate ideas for possible points of motivation during your weight loss journey.

- Do it for your family. This is a popular one, but it is popular because it is so important. If you are having trouble digging up the necessary motivation to do this for yourself, think about doing it for your family instead. If you lose weight and improve your health, it is almost certain you will have more to give your family on a daily basis. You should have more energy to play with your kids, and more focus when having conversations around the dinner table. By improving yourself, you can improve life for those around you in a very direct manner. Thinking about weight loss as something you can do for others just might be the push you need to get it done.

- Do it for your lifestyle. It is hard to argue that being overweight doesn't interfere with your lifestyle to some degree. Depending on the kinds of things you like to do, your weight may be getting in the way of enjoying some of your favorite activities, or it may be stopping you from keeping up with your friends. It would be a shame to go through life without being able to do your favorite things, simply because you were over-weight. Picture what your life might be like if you manage to get yourself down to a healthy weight – that image in your head may be all it takes to keep going on the path toward a healthy lifestyle.

- Do it for your career. Believe it or not, it is very possible that your weight is holding you back from advancing your career – even if your work requires nothing more physical than sitting at a desk. When you are overweight, it is likely that you'll struggle with energy during certain times of the day (such as the late afternoon lull we mentioned previously). If you fail to bring your full energy to the office day after day, you may get passed up for a promotion by other, more energetic employees. If you are someone who is driven by career achievement and advancement, you may be motivated by the thought of doing a favor to your professional life by successfully losing weight.

- Do it for your health. Staying motivated by this point alone is not going to work for everybody, but this is probably the most important reason of all to take your weight seriously. Carrying extra weight is bad for your health – it's just that simple. If you can successfully remove some of those extra pounds through a combination of a healthy diet and appropriate exercise, you should find yourself on a path toward improved overall health. Maintaining a healthy body weight is no guarantee of future health, of course, but it is a massive step in the right direction.

It is very possible that the ideal motivation for you is nowhere to be found on the list above. And that's okay – it is always going to be up to you in the end to find your own personal motivations to make it through this process. Your motivations need to be real, they need to be authentic, and they need to be powerful. Once you have the right motivation in mind, you just might be surprised to find how easy the rest of the task can be.

Positive Framing

When you embark on a mission to reduce your weight in a healthy manner, you need to see this journey in a positive frame of mind right from the start. This is absolutely critical. Most people, when they get started, see the combination of diet and exercise as a negative – it is something that they have to do in order to get healthy. Don't look at it that way. If at all possible, see this is an opportunity to improve yourself. Rather than seeing the process with a sense of dread, look forward to it as a way to make life better, one day at a time. This might seem like a small point, but it can actually make all of the difference in the world.

Pay attention to the way you talk about this process when telling family members or friends about what you are doing. You shouldn't be speaking of it in negative terms. Rather, you should be upbeat, positive, and excited. After all, think about what you have a chance to accomplish! You could make a positive change that can affect the rest of your life if you are able to stick with this process and move yourself to a healthy weight at some point in the near future. There is a lot to be excited about here.

If you've failed with your weight loss attempts in the past, as so many people have, we are willing to bet that those failures were at least in part related to your attitude about the process. It is crucial that you start with a great mindset, and you keep that mindset in a positive place while working toward your goals. Is every day going to be easy? Absolutely not. Are you going to think about giving up from time to time, or going back to your old ways? Of course. Don't be too hard on yourself when you have moments of weakness. Instead, continue to think positively, understand that this is a challenge, and turn your attitude around as soon as possible.

Remember that our mind and bodies are capable of achieving great and wonderful things and being focused on the right factors will help reveal our body's true potential.

This is Not a 'Diet'

To many people, the word 'diet' is one which belongs in the same category as many other four-letter words. And we tend to agree. Diets are usually made up of strict rules, odd food combinations, plenty of restrictions, and very little fun. There is a reason nearly every diet fails, and that is because they are unrealistic and not suited to real life.

So, instead of continuing to fail on diet after diet, you should instead just stop dieting altogether. We are not asking you to go on a diet – we are asking you to change your diet. There is a big difference. Instead of starting a diet with the intention of quitting it once you reach your goal weight, you can just change the way you eat and continue to eat that way with no end in sight.

At first, it is going to seem like a nearly impossible challenge to actually change the way you eat on a permanent basis. However, at some point along the way, a strange thing is likely to happen. Instead of forcing yourself to eat healthier foods like fruits and vegetables, you'll actually begin to crave them. Those unhealthy, processed foods you used to love won't sound good anymore, and you'll find yourself automatically filling your shopping basket with healthy options when you go to the grocery store. It is hard to see that future if you are reading this while overweight and on an unhealthy diet, but it really is a future that can be yours.

A Word on Enjoying Food

Before we wrap up this chapter on motivation, we want to touch quickly on the idea of that you have to give up enjoying your food when you start trying to lose weight. Nothing could be further from the truth. There are endless recipes available today for delicious, healthy meals that you can prepare at home. No matter what kinds of flavors you happen to enjoy, it will be easy to find healthy options that you can use to spice up your meals on a daily basis.

Eating bland, boring food isn't enjoyable for anyone. You don't want to stick yourself with a boring diet just because you need to lose weight. In fact, you are far more likely to succeed in the long run if you make sure your diet remains both healthy and exciting. You should be looking forward to dinner each night, not dreading the food that you have to consume. Pretty soon, you will have developed a long list of healthy recipes that you love to cook and eat with your family and friends. Moving forward, you can continue to love food just as you always have. Only now you'll be loving healthy foods, which you will find are actually much more satisfying in the end. You might have to spend a bit more time in the kitchen to prepare your meals – rather than just eating something from a box – but it will be worth it.

CHAPTER TEN

WRAPPING IT UP

At this point, we turn it over to you. What are you going to do next? Are you going to continue with the status quo, or are you going to make some changes? You know what the results are going to be if you keep up with your current habits – you will get the same results that you have been getting for years. If you are overweight now, maintaining your current diet and level of exercise is going to keep you overweight. If you think that somehow something is going to change without you taking direct action, you are lying to yourself.

One of the keys to having success with your weight loss goals is to understand that you don't have to win the entire battle in a single day. If you have bad habits with regard to your diet, for instance, those habits aren't going to change overnight. It took years to create your current patterns, and it will take some time – and effort – to undo them. Rather than trying to overcome every single mistake all at once, start with some small goals and go from there.

With this concept in mind, let's take a look at a few examples of how you can break your weight loss mission down into some smaller first steps.

- Give up one vice. To make some progress on your diet, try starting by sacrificing one of your unhealthy vices. For instance, if you regularly consume soft drinks, try eliminating those from your diet – or at least cut back on how many you drink per day or try replacing it for soda water. The challenge of getting rid of one vice won't be an easy one, but it should be manageable. Once that is done and you are happy with your progress, you can set your sights on another milestone. As you keep checking off positive changes, you will soon have dramatically shifted your dietary habits.

- Make a fruits and veggies swap. Even if you aren't ready to overhaul your entire diet, try just switching out some of your daily foods for fresh fruits and veggies. For example, try trading out some processed food that you would have used as a side dish (chips, potatoes, pasta) for dinner with some fresh veggies. Or, toss out that candy bar you were going to eat as a snack and consume an apple or orange instead. Starting with some of these basic swaps is a good way to make gradual progress. If you can keep making more and more of these healthy trades throughout the day, your diet is quickly going to round into shape.

• Add incidental exercise. Adding exercise to your daily routine doesn't have to be as dramatic as joining a gym and sweating heavily for long periods of time. To get started, try adding 'incidental' exercise to your day to day routine. As long as it is okay with your doctor, and within the limits of your health, change some of your basic habits. Try taking the stairs at work instead of riding the elevator. Park your car farther away from the building to make your walk a little longer. These kinds of changes might not seem significant, and they aren't when you view them individually, but taken together they represent a big step toward improved fitness.

As you can see, it doesn't have to be daunting to start taking steps toward a healthier, lighter you. With that said, nothing is going to happen if you don't take action. It's easy to keep thinking about doing it later, like next Monday, or next week, or next month. Those thoughts might make you feel good for a moment, but they aren't actually going to allow you to accomplish anything. Replace your thoughts with action steps that will lead your health and your weight toward the I.D.E.A.L you.

Thank you for taking the time to read this book. We hope the information contained throughout will help you work successfully toward your weight loss goals. Remember, always be smart when it comes to your health, and talk to your doctor before making any changes. You can do this, but it isn't always going to be easy. Find your motivation, create a plan, and execute on that plan one day at a time. Good luck!

www.ingramcontent.com/pod-product-compliance
Lightning Source LLC
Chambersburg PA
CBHW070809240726
48654CB00007B/273